Simplified Yoga

for

Backache

By Subodh Gupta

Corporate Yoga Trainer

First Edition March 2008

ISBN 978-0-9556882-4-9

Published by
Subodh Gupta
+44(0)7966275913
Headquarter: London (UK)
Email: info@subodhgupta.com
www.subodhgupta.com

Publisher Note:

The reader should not regard the recommendations and Yoga exercises expressed and described in this book as substitute advice of a qualified medical practitioner. It is also advisable that reader may learn the Yoga exercises initially in presence of a qualified yoga trainer.

Acknowledgements

I am grateful to my parents and all my teachers who taught me at various stages of my life & shared with me their wisdom.

I am also thankful to Models: Zosia Lesiecka, Duncan Hogg and Barbara Tomasik for taking their time out of their busy schedule to help me to complete my book.

Content

Part 3:

Introduction:

This book is a practical guide on preventing and managing back pain. It is based on my own experience while teaching Yoga.

People most often suffer from lower back, shoulder and neck pain for various reasons, for example: during long hours of sitting at a workstation, working in front of a computer, driving long distances, gardening, lifting a small child from the floor, stress, etc.

There are other reasons as well which can be responsible for our backache, for example: one may fall down or because of an accident or pregnancy but majority of back pain cases happen because of a weak and inflexible back.

A strong and flexible back creates the foundation for a healthy lifestyle.

Our back bears almost all of our body weight and any extra weight we carry. If our back is not healthy we cannot be healthy.

Backache can be avoided or at least minimised in the first place if our back is strong and flexible.

Yoga poses described in this book will not only strengthen the back muscles and bring flexibility to our back but will also help in reducing stress. Simplified yoga postures described in this book can be practiced by everybody, whether young or old, beginner or advanced.

This book consists of 3 parts. First part of the book contains understanding about back pain, how it affects our body, its prevention and the benefits of yoga. Second part is about simplified yoga exercises for flexibility, strength and reducing stress. The third part is to record your yoga practice and improvement in your lower back, shoulders and neck.

In the end I would like to say that practicing Yoga should be pleasant and enjoyable. *If you do it regularly, gently with breath awareness in your daily life, you can enjoy your work and life without getting injured.*

May all being be healthy.

Subodh Gupta

Part 1

Understanding about Back Pain

A strong and flexible back creates the foundation for a healthy lifestyle.

About Back Pain

Back pain is very common and is one of the most frequent complaints among people. According to a survey published in 2000 *almost half the adult population of the UK (49%) report low back pain lasting for at least 24 hours at some time in the year.*[1] *31 million Americans experience low-back pain at any given time.*[2]

Our back is a very complex network of bones, joints, muscles, tendons and ligaments and back pain can happen because of any of them getting injured.

The pain can be felt constantly or intermittently. The pain may be felt in the lower back or may radiate into a leg or a foot.

Most cases of back pain are not caused by serious conditions such as infection, bone fracture, chronic constipation, etc. *In general back pain lasts for a couple of days and can be corrected by taking rest.* However, if the pain persists it is necessary that one should see a doctor.

Why majority of back pain happens in the lumbar spine (lower back)?

Because the lumbar spine bears most of our body weight and any extra weight which we lift that's why majority of back pain happens here.

Causes of back pain?

There is no single reason for back pain and often it is difficult to determine the real cause.

Back pain can be triggered by any of the following activities at home, work, play, during driving *due to poor posture*:

- Lifting or pulling incorrectly,
- Slouching in a chair,
- Bending down for long period of time,
- Twisting during golf,
- Muscle tension,
- Continuous driving for long period.

Some other causes of back pain are:

- Pregnancy,
- Stress ,
- Kidney infections,
- Osteoporosis,
- Fall,
- Fracture,
- Weak back muscles,
- Chronic constipation,
- Obesity

Back pain in the corporate organizations

Back pain is one of the most common reasons for missed work. *British business loses an estimated 4.9 million days to employee absenteeism through work-related back conditions each year, with each affected employee taking an average of 19 days off work, according to the latest figures from the 2003/4 Labour Force Survey.*[3] *Americans spend at least $50 billion each year on back pain.*[2]

Reasons for Back Pain: The most common reasons for back pain in corporate houses are: *Poor Posture* (both sitting and standing), *Sedentary Lifestyle* and *excessive Stress.*

The problem of back pain is further aggravated because of the inflexibility and muscular insufficiency in the muscles.

Bad Sitting Posture:

In my opinion this is the single most important factor which causes back pain to the corporate executives. Let's see how:

Corporate executives work in their offices for an average *8 hours a day* in a sitting position; travelling to the office and back home take additional 2 *hours* sitting while driving; time spend in eating breakfast, lunch, dinner add another 1 hour of sitting; watching baseball or football or cricket on TV takes additional 1 hour.

So if we calculate the total time spent in all the above activities, we can clearly see that the *executives spend about 12 hours out of 24 hours (50% time) only in a sitting position. Now imagine what would happen if the sitting posture is not correct?*

Believe it or not after seeing many of the offices computer workstation, I can say with conviction that there is hardly any consideration given while designing the offices furniture to keep our back healthy.

So analysis is, sitting posture is the most important parameter to consider while planning your backache management plan as executives spend about 12 hours out of 24 hours (50% time) only in a sitting position.

Sedentary Lifestyle:

Technology has made our life easy but has also made our lifestyle sedentary. It is the regular physical activity which keeps our muscles strong, and lack of it will weaken the muscles.

Excessive Stress:

Excessive Stress is also one of the major reasons for back pain as there is a strong connection between stress and back pain.

Stress hormones cause the muscles to tighten up and muscle tension reduces blood flow to the tissues (reduced oxygen and nutrients to the tissues) which delay healing process.

The back is less capable of tolerating even mild abuse (lifting something slightly heavy, sitting too long, etc) when a person is under stress.

Stress causes the muscles to tighten up, leaving them more vulnerable to injury. By reducing Stress one can reduce pain which is aggravated or caused by tense muscles.

Managing stress on a regular basis can help in preventing back pain from occurring in the first place.

Corporate executives face all the major problems by virtue of their job. Their lifestyle is sedentary, have wrong sitting posture during long working hours and lots of stressful work, hence the backache.

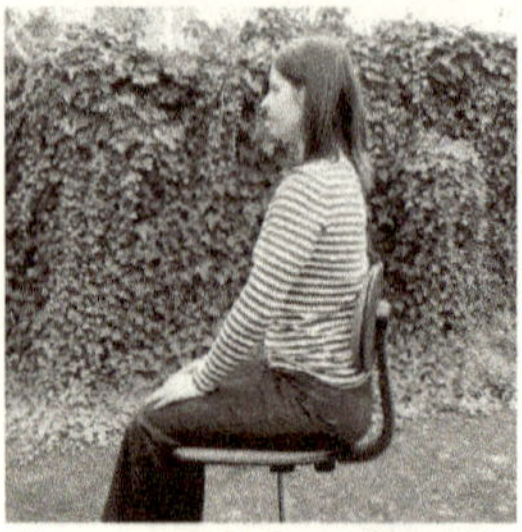
Correct Sitting Position

(Back Straight is safe)

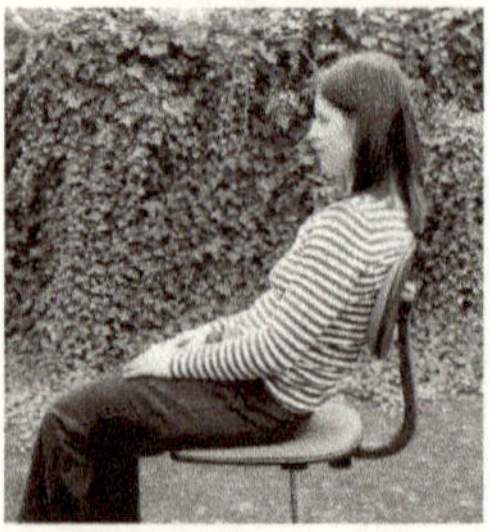
Incorrect Sitting Position

(Slouching on a chair can hurt your back over a period of time)

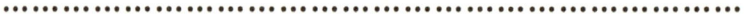

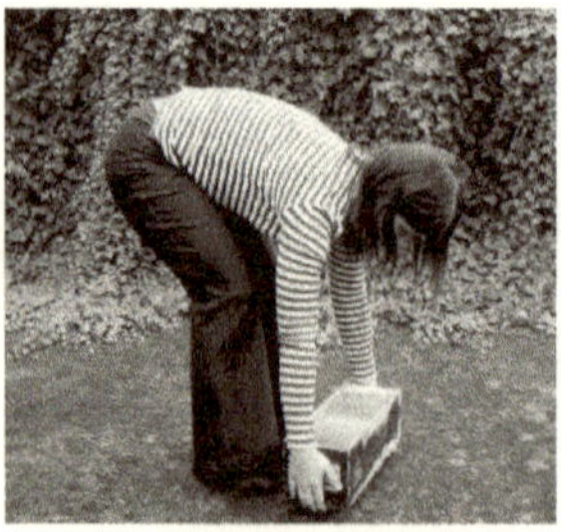
Safe Lifting position
(Knees bent, so back is safe)

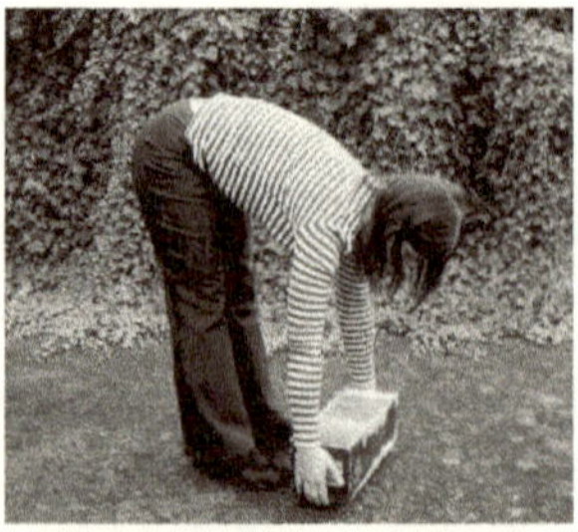
Unsafe lifting position
(Straight Knees, more chances of back injury)

Prevention and Effective Management of Backache:

Following 2 steps would help you in both preventing and managing your backache.

Step No 1: Prevention Tips

Learn the right posture for yourself while sitting, driving, lifting, standing, playing, etc. For example:

-Adjust your work station height *so your back is straight without any discomfort* or you may need to change your chair at the office or adjust its height.

-Adjust your car seat or you may need to use a support (small pillow).

-Bend your knees while lifting anything from the floor.

-If you are on long drive then take breaks; get out of the car and stretch during journey.

-Wear comfortable and low-heel shoes because high heels push the pelvis forward stressing the lumbar spine.

-Quit smoking. It is always a good idea to quit smoking if you are having back pain as smoking impairs blood flow which results in less oxygen and nutrients to the spinal tissues.

Sitting posture is the most important parameter to consider while planning your backache management plan as executives spend about 12 hours out of 24 hours (50 % time) only in a sitting position.

-Drink at least 8 glasses of water a day.

-Lose any excess weight if you think that you are having excess body weight. Not only will it help you to protect your back but also your knees.

Step No 2: Developing Strength, Flexibility and relieving Stress

If sufficient muscular strength is build up along with flexibility the chances of back pain can always be minimised. One needs active lifestyle and along with it one can follow the Yoga exercise plan which I have designed to achieve a strong and flexible back.

Simplified yoga exercises explained below are gentle and will help to bring flexibility and strength to your back muscles. They are also excellent for releasing Stress hence perfect for both prevention and managing backache.

General solution is to take bed rest as soon as possible if you feel backache.

Bed should not be too cushy. In fact I would recommend a thin mattress (*good enough to provide cushion for your spine from hard base*) over plain and hard wooden base.

Yoga poses should be practiced every day for about 15 to 20 minutes if you want to live a life which is free from backache. Yoga poses will certainly help to increase the muscular strength of various muscles group apart from bringing flexibility to the body's joints and muscles.

Daily 15 min yoga exercises plan for Healthy Back.

I would recommend that you may practice from exercise no 1 to 11 every day if you really want to keep your back healthy and minimise the chances of lower back and neck pain.

Notes for Yoga Practitioners

Breathing through Nose or Mouth: Always breathe through the nose with the awareness (unless specified by mouth). *Remember a simple concept that by nature, mouth is for eating and nose is for breathing.* Please do not try to reverse the nature functions. As you breathe in, know that you are breathing in. As you breathe out, know that you are breathing out. This will greatly enhance your general health and well-being.

Nose performs not only the breathing function but it filters the air, moisturise the air, warms the air, it can smell, it secretes the mucus and performs many more functions.

Now think for a moment if the mouth can perform all these functions..

Yes you are thinking correctly, mouth cannot perform all these functions, so please do not breathe through mouth unless specified in some special exercises.

Place of Practice: It is good to practice in a room which is well ventilated. Please do not practice under a fan or direct sunlight.

Sitting Posture for Yoga: Any comfortable sitting position is ok. The main point is the body needs to be relaxed and back straight. Do not slump and do not lean forward. It is good to sit on a folded blanket or a cloth which is made of natural fibre.

In case if you find it difficult to sit on the floor in a cross leg sitting position, some of the yoga postures described in this book can also be practiced while sitting on the chair.

Relaxation: Whenever you feel tired during the practice of yoga exercises, lie down on the floor on your back for 2 - 3 minutes and try to relax.

Practice Time of Yoga: The best time for yoga practice is early morning during sunrise or around sunset (Yoga exercise should only be done after at least 3 hours of eating the food. For example if you want to do yoga exercise at 6pm in the evening then please make sure that your lunch should have been eaten by 3pm).

Awareness during Yoga: It is very important that while practicing yoga exercises you are aware of your breath and your body movement.

Any yoga posture without awareness of breath is a practice of a beginner.

Frequency of Practice: In my view yoga exercises should be practiced every day, however if not possible then at least 4 days a week.

Cautions: If you are suffering from any neck related pain, injury, hernia pain or have gone through any recent operation, please consult your doctor first before beginning any of the yoga exercises.

Please Note: This Yoga book is strictly **not for women** who are **going through pregnancy**. In case of pregnancy I would recommend that you may please consult an experienced personal yoga trainer only.

Part 2

15 Minutes Daily Yoga Plan

All the yoga poses described in this book are carefully selected for managing backache. However if you experience any discomfort while practicing any of the yoga poses please avoid that pose.

15 Minutes Yoga Exercises Plan

Exercise 1

Neck: Forward and Back Bend

Preparation: Sit in a cross-legged position on the floor with hands resting on your knees and back straight (*You can also sit on the chair with your back straight if you find sitting on the floor with cross leg position inconvenient to you*).

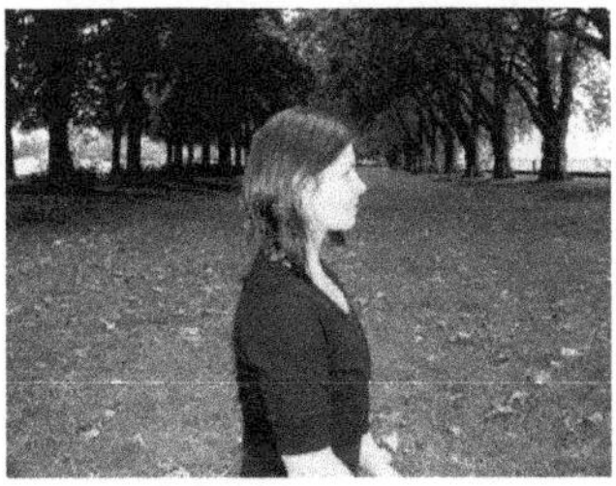

Caution: There should not be any strain in any neck movement. You can take your head forward and back only to the point where you feel absolutely comfortable.

Step1: As you exhale slowly bring your head down.

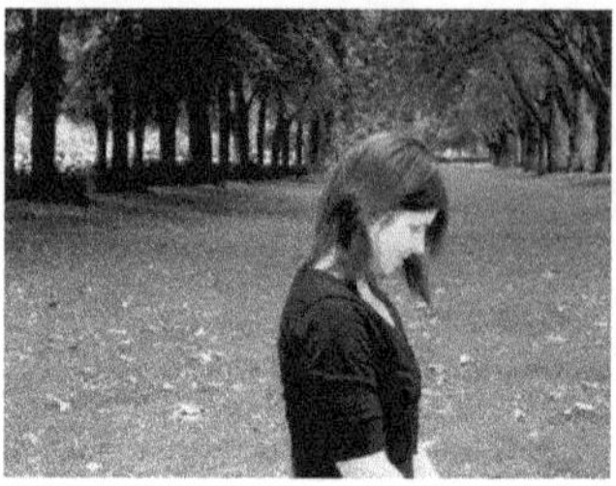

Step2: As you inhale move your head back as far as you feel comfortable.

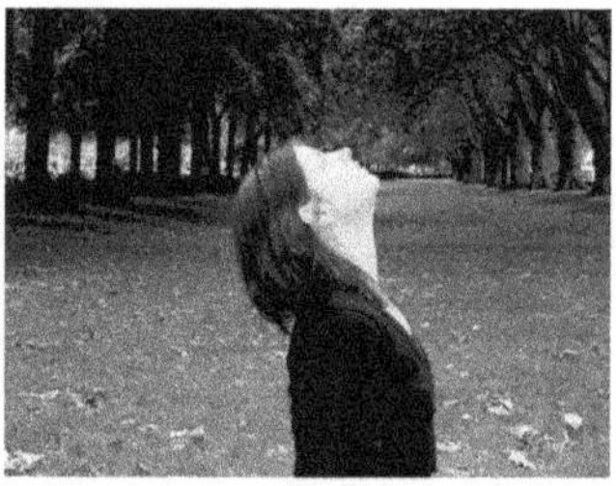

This is one round.

Practice 5 rounds.

Exercise2

Neck: Chin over shoulder

Preparation: Sit in a cross-legged position with hands resting on your knees with back straight.

Step1: As you exhale turn your head towards your right shoulder.

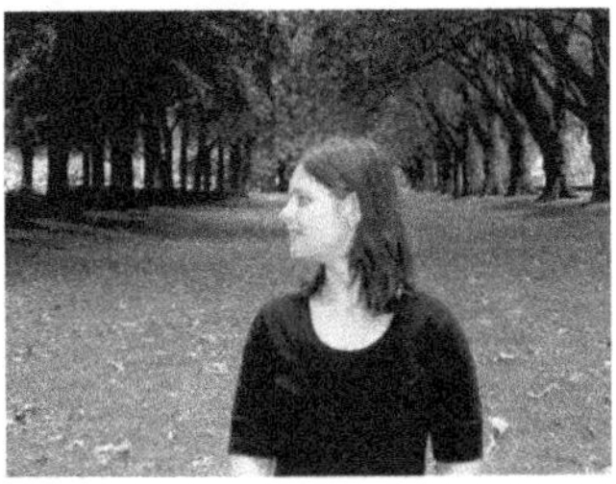

Step2: Inhale and bring the head to the centre position.

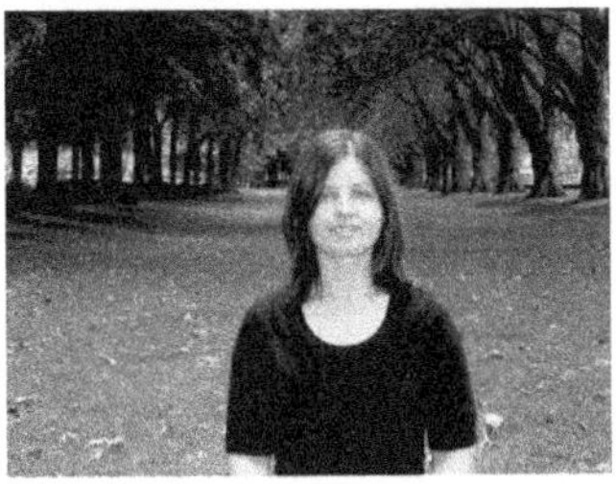

Step3: As you exhale turn your head towards your left shoulder.

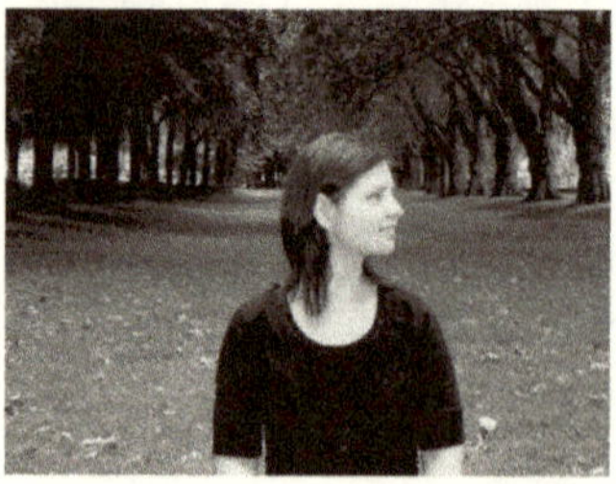

Step4: Inhale and bring the head to the centre.

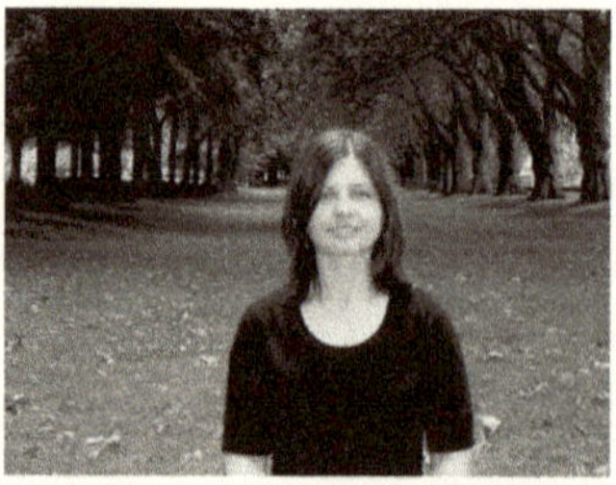

This is one round.

Practice 5 rounds.

Exercise 3

Neck: Ear to Shoulder movement

Preparation: Sit in a cross-legged pose with hands resting on your knees with back straight.

Step1: As you exhale lower your head toward your right shoulder (lowering right ear towards your right shoulder as shown in the picture).

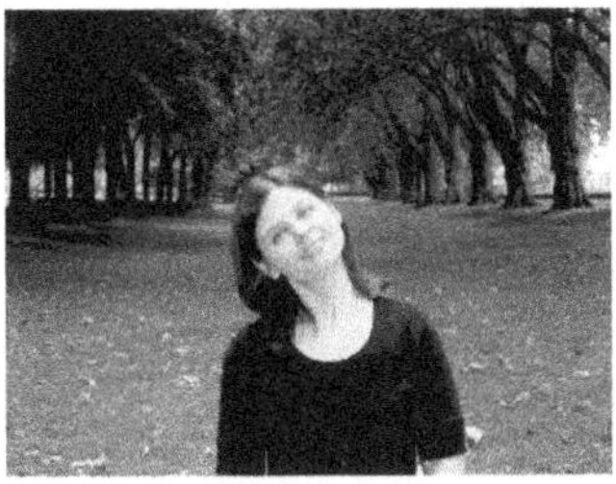

Step2: Inhale and come back to the centre.

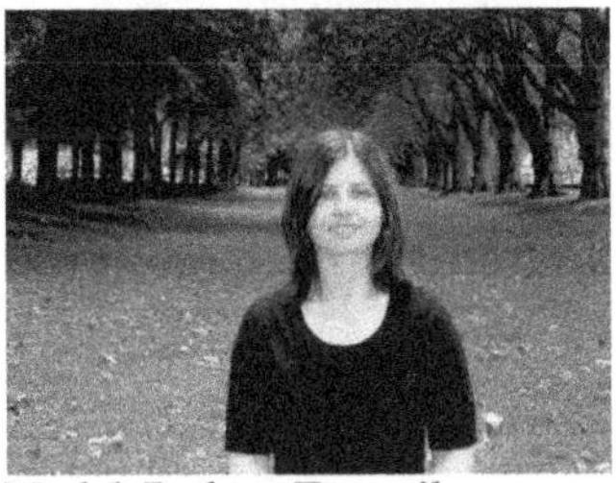

Model: Barbara Tomasik

Step3: As you exhale lower your head toward your left shoulder.

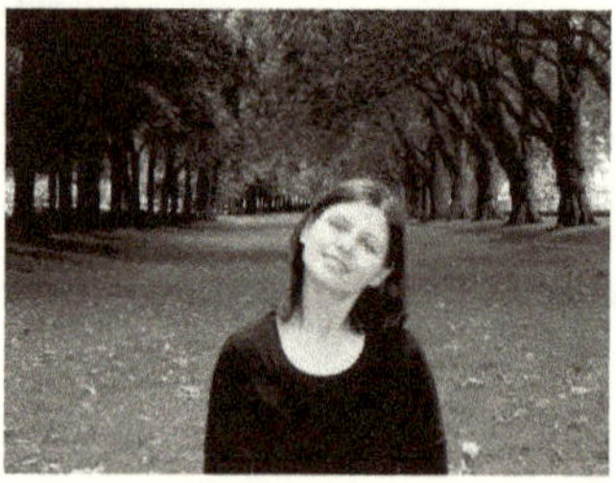

Step4: Inhale and come back to the centre (these all steps complete one round).

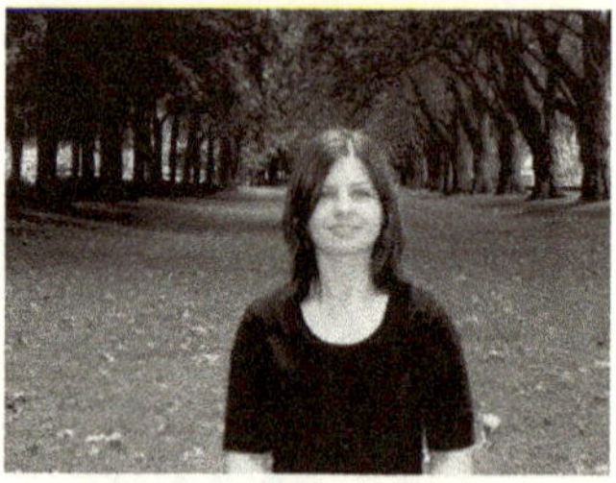

Practice 5 rounds.

Benefits:

These 3 neck exercises release tension and stiffness in the head, neck and shoulders, especially after prolonged work at the desk.

Precautions:

If you are suffering from any kind of neck related pain, injury or cervical spondylosis, please consult your doctor first before beginning any of the gentle neck exercises.

Note: *The shoulders should not move in any of the neck exercises. Please be aware while practicing neck movements that only the neck and head should move.*

Exercise 4
Shoulder Rotation

Preparation: Sit in a crossed-legged position on the floor with your back straight (*or you may sit on the chair with your back straight if you find it difficult to sit on the floor*).

Place your fingers on your shoulders with elbows down.

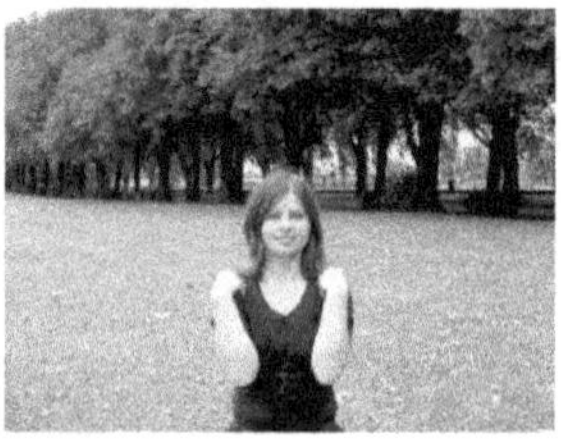

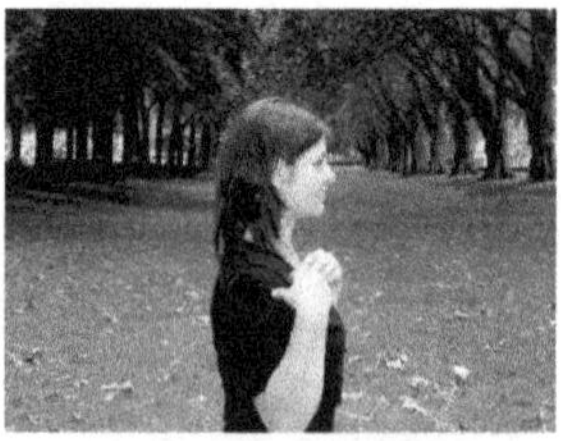

Step1: As you inhale rotate your shoulders upward (*elbows going up towards the ceiling as shown in the picture below*).

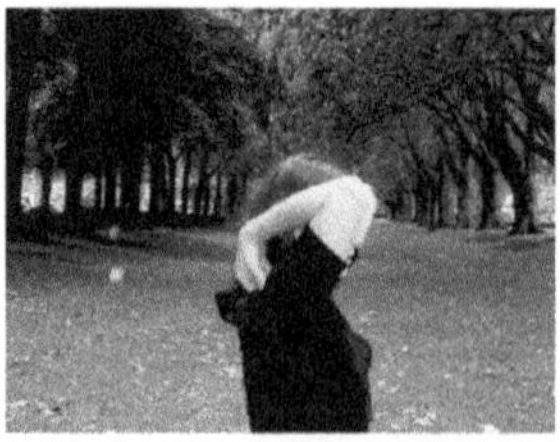

Step2: As you exhale fully rotate your shoulders downward (elbows going down towards the floor as shown in picture below).

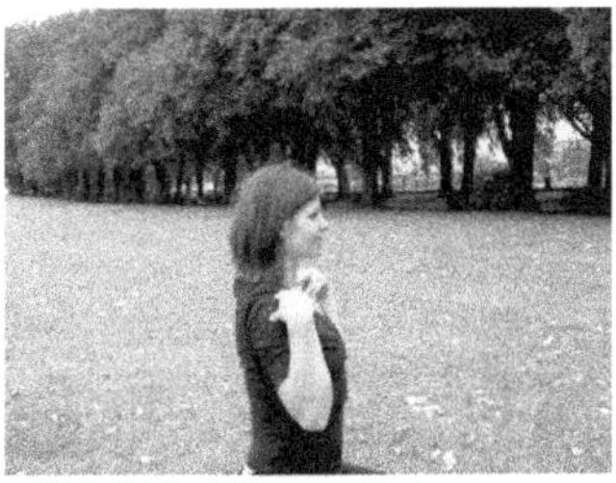

This completes one round.

Practice 5 rounds clockwise and 5 rounds anticlockwise.

Benefits:

This shoulder movement releases the strain of driving, long hours of office work and also helps in bringing mobility to tight shoulders.

Exercise 5

Cat Stretch

Come up in a position as shown in the picture below with your knees under your hips and your palms under your shoulders.

Your wrists, elbows and shoulders are in line and perpendicular to the floor. Centre your head in a neutral position, eyes looking at the floor (picture below).

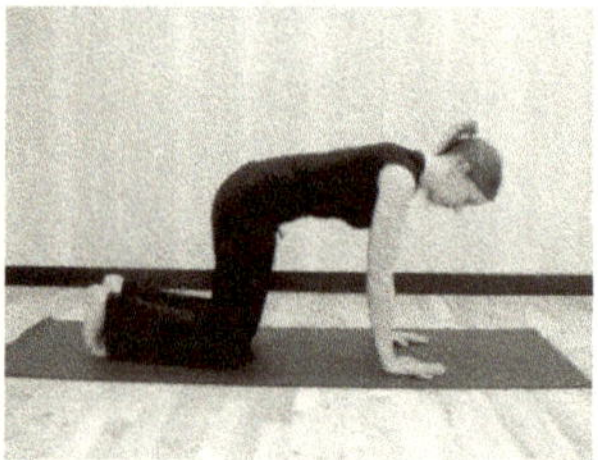

While inhaling slowly and deeply, lift your head up and bring your spine down within your comfort level as shown in the picture below.

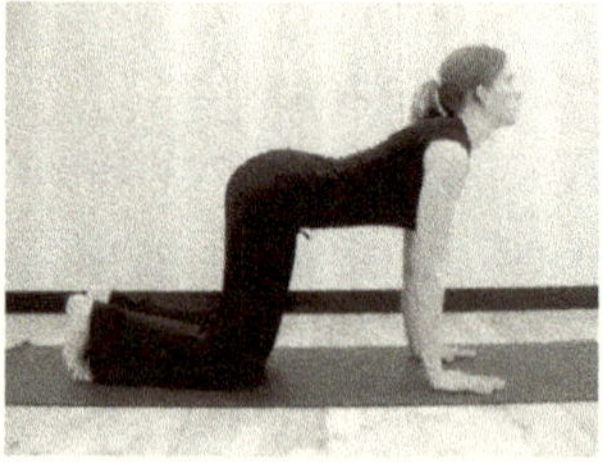

As you slowly exhale bring you head down and round your spine toward the ceiling and contract your abdomen as shown in the picture below.

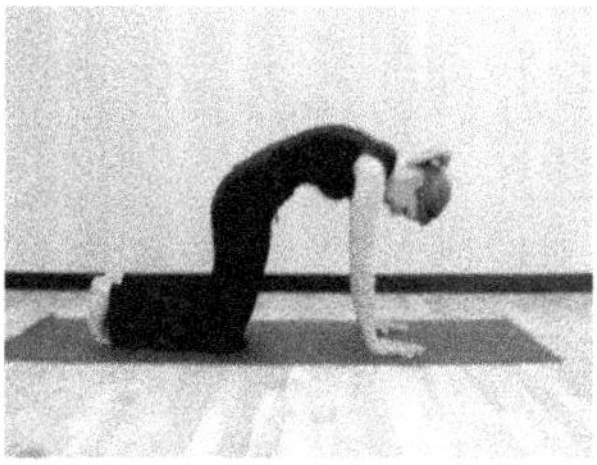

This inhalation and exhalation complete one round. You can practice 5 to 10 rounds.

This is a very good exercise for improving flexibility of the spine and it is especially helpful after long hours of sitting in the office or driving to release stiffness from the back.

Caution:

In case of neck injury and pregnancy, please practice it under guidance of an experienced yoga teacher only.

Exercise 6

Cycling Exercise

Step 1: Lie down on your back and slowly lift your both legs up as shown in the picture.

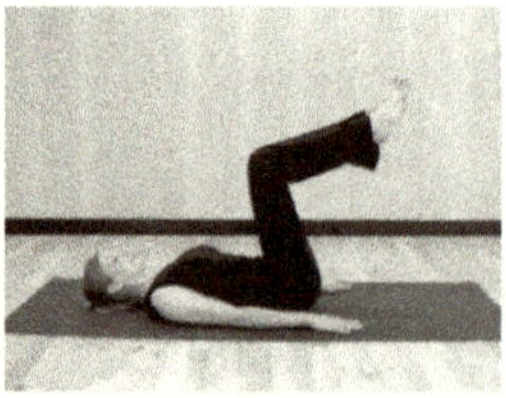

Step 2: Now start moving your legs as you do while cycling and practice 10 cycles in forward direction.

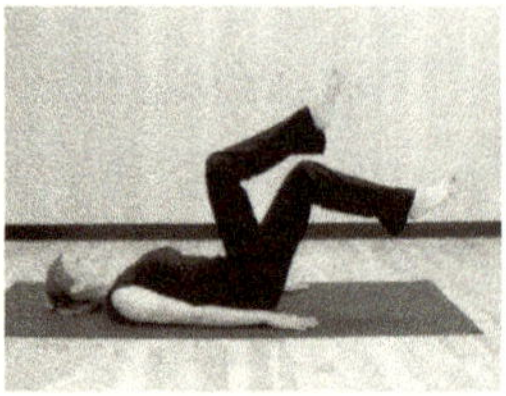

Step 3: After completing 10 cycles in forward direction, make another 10 circles in reverse direction.

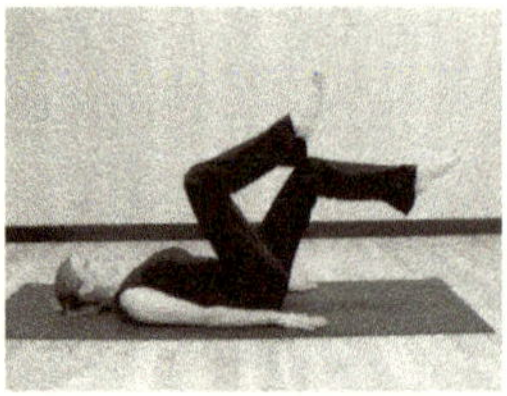

Step 4: Bring your feet down on the floor with your knees bent and relax for the next 30 seconds.

Benefits: This is another good exercise for abs and lower back muscles.

Note:

(1) Cycling movement should be slow.

(2) Gradually you can increase the number of cycling counts to 15 and then 20 depending upon your own comfort level. (*Never force yourself or strain yourself while practicing Yoga exercises*).

(3) If your *lower back is weak* then please make cycling movement in a **small circle**.

Exercise 7

Single Leg Lock pose

Step by step method:

Step 1: Lie down on your back on the floor with your right knee bent towards the chest and keep your left leg relaxed and straight.

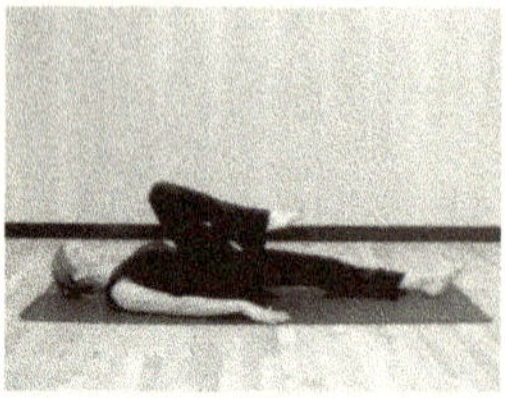

Step2: Interlock your fingers below the right knee.

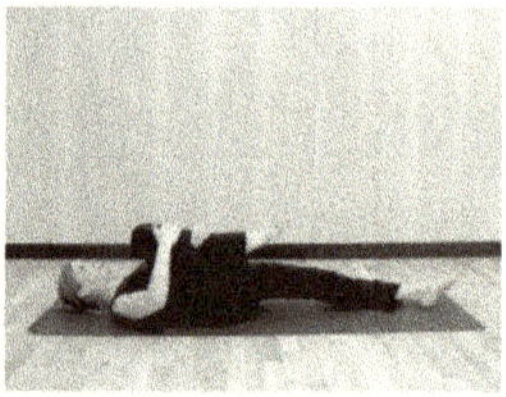

Step 3: First inhale deeply in lying position and then **while exhaling,** slowly raise your head or your chin up towards your right knee.

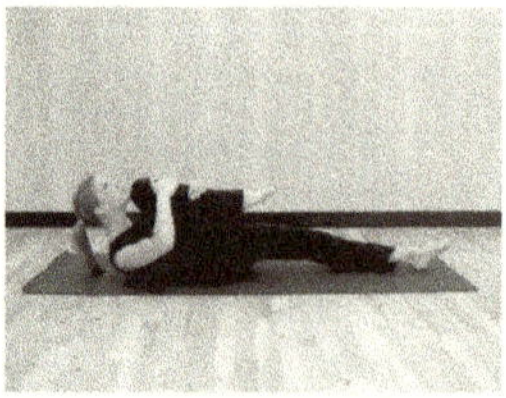

(*Raise your head or chin towards your right knee to the point where you feel comfortable*).

Step 4: Now **while inhaling,** slowly come down to lying position.

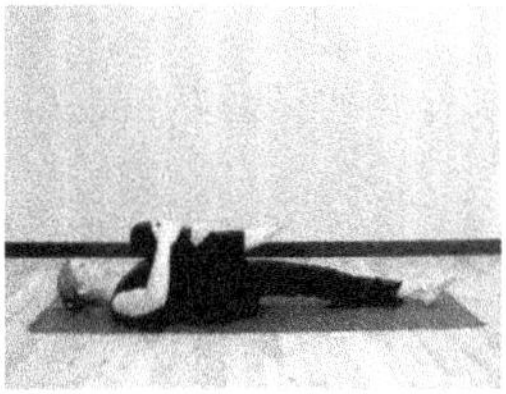

Release the right knee and repeat the same with your left leg. This will complete one round.

Practice 3 - 6 rounds.

Benefits:

It is very effective in removing unwanted wind from the body.

It is also helpful in removing constipation.

Precautions: People suffering from slipped disc or sciatica should avoid this posture or consult an experienced yoga teacher before practicing the pose.

Exercise 8

Spinal Twist

Step by step method:

Preparation: Lie flat on your back with your legs straight and palms facing down.

Step 1: Bend the right knee and place the right foot on the floor by the left knee.

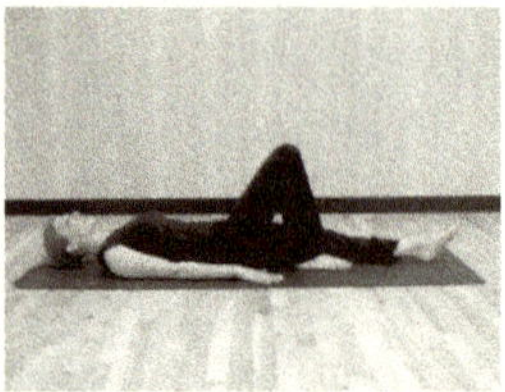

Then place your left hand on top of the right knee, as shown in picture.

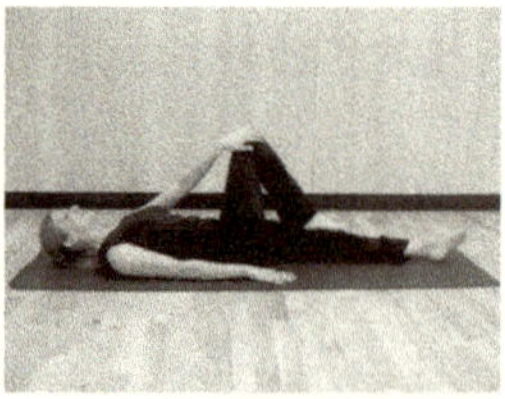

Step 2: As you exhale, bring your right knee down towards the floor on the left side of your body, turning around 45 degree left side or half way and turn your head to the right side of your body.

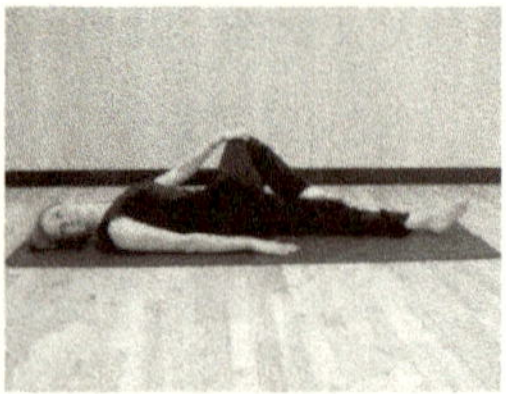

(Note: *In this position your right arm and your right shoulder should be touching the floor comfortably*).

Now hold this posture for about 30 seconds and keep breathing naturally.

Step 3: As you inhale slowly return to the centre.

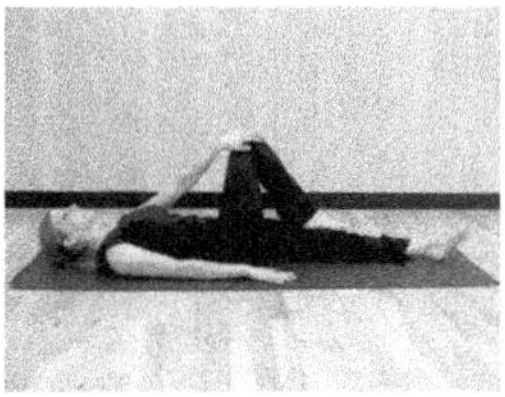

Step 4: Repeat on the other side (this completes one round).

Benefits: This yoga posture helps in releasing tightness and tiredness in the lower back and it is excellent for you, if you have a job which involves sitting on the chair for long hours.

Caution: If you experience pain at any stage, please make sure that you are not overstretching.

Exercise 9

Cobra pose

In this backbend yoga pose you lift upper part of the body away from the floor against the gravity and return to the starting position with the help of gravity.

Breathing:
Inhale - while rising up
Breathe normally while holding the pose
Exhale - while lowering down

Step by step method:

Step 1: Lie flat on the stomach with legs straight, heels and toes together. Place your hands alongside the chest, with the palms down and the elbows close to your body and rest the forehead on the floor.

Step 2: Inhale and slowly lift your forehead, neck and chest of the floor looking up. (Remember to lift your upper body up mainly using your back and neck muscles).

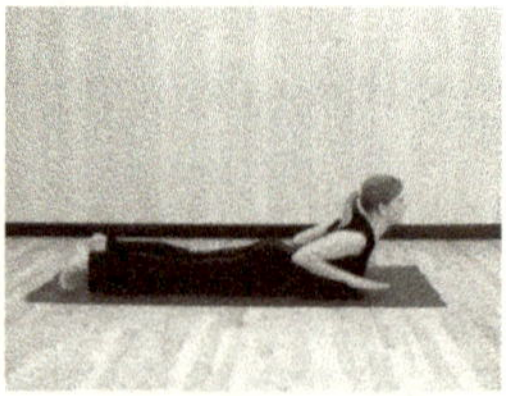

Step 3: Once you come up hold this posture and breathe normally. Please do not put much weight on your palms. Stay in this posture initially for 2 to 3 breaths.

Step 4: While exhaling gently come down.

Gradually you can increase the holding time of cobra posture up to 10 breaths as you feel more comfortable.

Benefits:

It helps to reduce backache.

It keeps the spine supple and healthy.

It helps alleviate constipation.

It stimulates the appetite.

Precautions:

People suffering from *hernia, peptic ulcer, and intestinal tuberculosis should not practice* this pose without expert guidance.

Pregnant women should not practice this yoga pose at all.

Common Mistakes:

Students use more of the arm muscles than their back muscles.

Students straighten their arms and tense their shoulders.

Note:

I have seen many times that beginners try cobra posture as shown in the picture below and also in some of the yoga classes yoga teachers are encouraging students to practice this kind of yoga position.

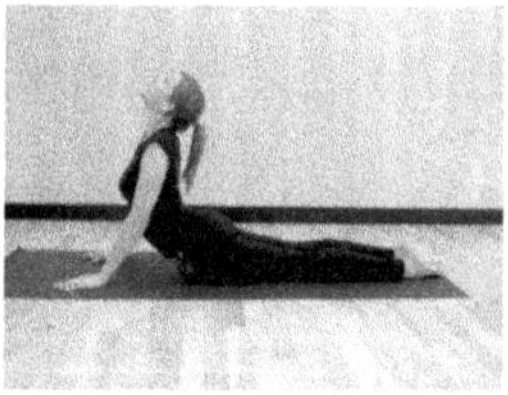

(This yoga position is not suitable for most of the people)

This position would certainly create backache and injure those people whose back is stiff and I would strongly advise not to practice this position.

Exercise 10

Child's pose

This yoga posture stretches the spine from end to end and it is relaxing, refreshing and calming.

Breathing:

Inhale - while raising the arms above the head
Exhale - while bending forward
Breathe normally while relaxing in the pose.

Step by step method:

1.Sit on your heals, placing your palms on the thighs above the knees, keeping your spine and head straight as shown in the picture below.

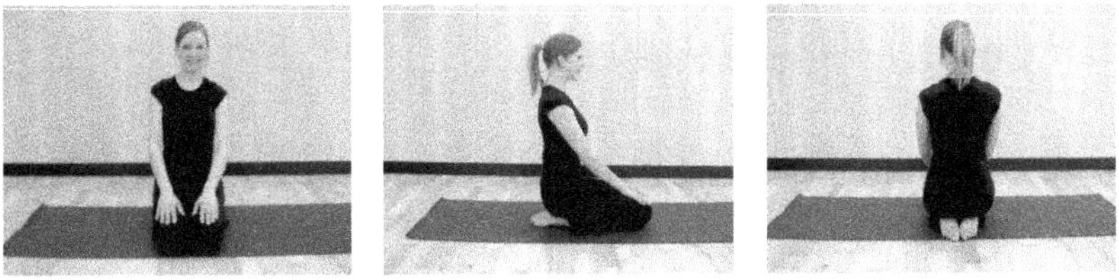

Model: Zosia Lesiecka

(If you find difficulty sitting on your heals as shown in picture you may place small pillow under your ankles).

2. Inhale while raising your arms above the head.

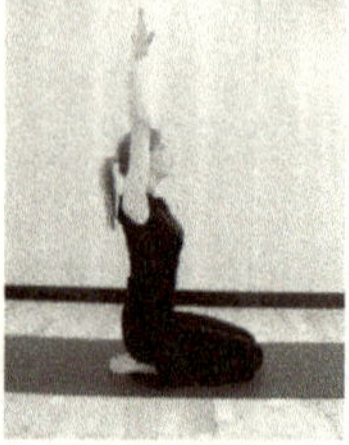

3. Bend forward while exhaling. Rest your forehead on the floor in front of your knees, and your arms alongside the legs, with the palms up.

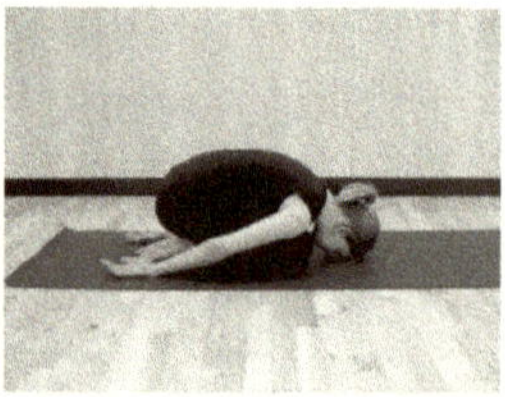

If you are a beginner, stay in this posture for about 30 seconds and later on gradually increase to 3 minutes.

Benefits:

1. It stretches the back muscles.

2. It tones the pelvic muscles.

3. It helps to relieves constipation.

Note:

If you find difficult to breathe in the child's pose then keep your knees apart.

Precautions:

This posture should not be done in case of:

(a) Pregnancy (unless modified)

(b) Diarrhoea

(c) Knee injury

(d) Vertigo

Exercise 11

Simple Breathing Technique for Stress Release

Abdominal Breathing

Abdominal breathing is the most natural and efficient breathing. One can observe a little baby breath since the moment of his/her birth and it is abdominal breathing (also known as diaphragmatic breathing).

In this breathing exercise during inhalation abdomen moves up and during exhalation the abdomen moves down.

For performing abdominal breathing

First lie down flat on your back with your knees bend as shown in the picture below.

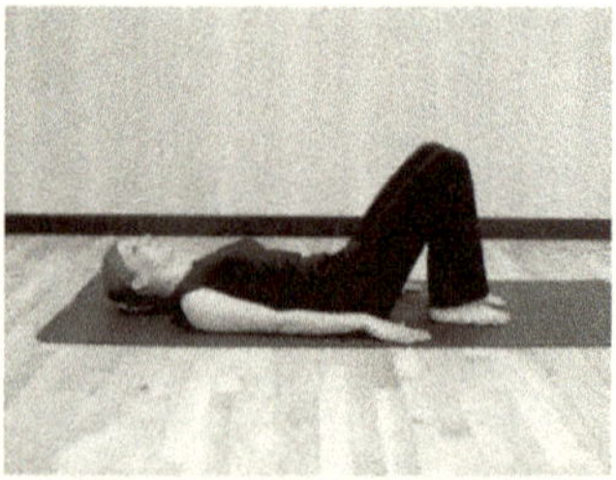

Knees Bend with Feet 6 inch Apart

Relax your whole body. Now place your left hand on the abdomen on your navel area.

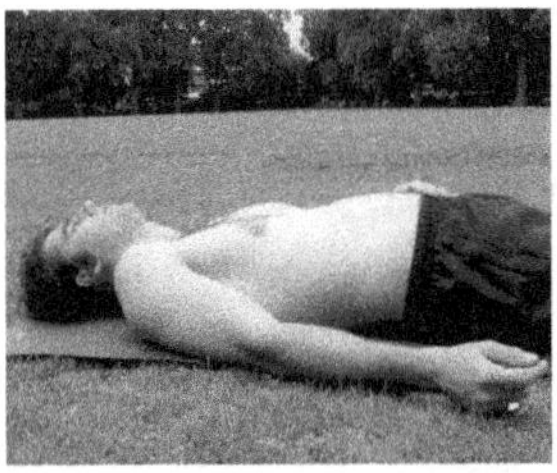

(**Abdomen position during inhalation)**

If you are breathing naturally through your abdomen, your left hand would move up with each inhalation and down with exhalation.

Try to take your breath **slowly** and **deeply**. The **slow, deep** and **smooth breath** would bring relaxation to the body and mind and release stress which is also one of the main reason for back pain. You can practice it at least 2 to 3 minutes every day with your yoga plan at the end of each yoga session.

Cautions:

Make sure that there are no jerks in the flow of your breath. The flow of your breath should be smooth and without any noise.

Part 3

Back Pain History

Write the information below in detail to help you remember what caused you back pain. *By referring to this information you may be able to avoid the activity which cause you pain.*

When did your back pain start?

What were you doing when the pain started?

Location of the pain.

Does the pain stay in the same place?

What makes the pain better, or worse?

Wellness Monitor

Before beginning yoga exercise plan, please take couple of minutes to fill in the following wellness monitor.

	Wellness Monitor	
S.N.	Indicators	Before Beginning
1	Blood Pressure (High)	
	(Low)	
2	Lower back pain	
3	Shoulder Pain	
4	Neck Pain	
5	Quality of sleep (1 to 5) (1 lowest and 5 the best, average for the week)	
6	Stress level (1 to 5) (1 lowest and 5 highest, average for the week)	
7	Overall energy level (1 to 5) (1 lowest and 5 highest)	

Yoga Practice Record

I would like to recommend that for your good health please practice yoga every day and after the practice mark your progress in the record below.

Starting date ....

Week 1	Sun	Mon	Tue	Wed	Thu	Fri	Sat
Yoga Practice							
Week 2	Sun	Mon	Tue	Wed	Thu	Fri	Sat
Yoga Practice							
Week 3	Sun	Mon	Tue	Wed	Thu	Fri	Sat
Yoga Practice							
Week 4	Sun	Mon	Tue	Wed	Thu	Fri	Sat
Yoga Practice							

After week 4 what improvement do you feel, please write in the box below

Wellness Monitor

Now you have completed 4 week yoga practice, please take couple of minutes to fill in the following wellness monitor.

	Wellness Monitor	
S.N.	Indicators	After 4 weeks
1	Blood Pressure (High)	
	(Low)	
2	Lower back pain	
3	Shoulder Pain	
4	Neck Pain	
5	Quality of sleep (1 to 5) (1 lowest and 5 the best, average for the week)	
6	Stress level (1 to 5) (1 lowest and 5 highest, average for the week)	
7	Overall energy level (1 to 5) (1 lowest and 5 highest)	

Yoga Practice Record

Please practice yoga every day and after the practice mark your progress in the record below.

Practice record Week 5 to 8

Week 5	Sun	Mon	Tue	Wed	Thu	Fri	Sat
Yoga Practice							
Week 6	Sun	Mon	Tue	Wed	Thu	Fri	Sat
Yoga Practice							
Week 7	Sun	Mon	Tue	Wed	Thu	Fri	Sat
Yoga Practice							
Week 8	Sun	Mon	Tue	Wed	Thu	Fri	Sat
Yoga Practice							

After week 8 what improvement do you feel, please write in the box below

Wellness Monitor

Now you have completed 8 week of yoga practice, please take couple of minutes to fill in the following wellness monitor.

	Wellness Monitor	
S.N.	Indicators	After 8 week
1	Blood Pressure (High)	
	(Low)	
2	Lower back pain	
3	Shoulder Pain	
4	Neck Pain	
5	Quality of sleep (1 to 5) (1 lowest and 5 the best, average for the week)	
6	Stress level (1 to 5) (1 lowest and 5 highest, average for the week)	
7	Overall energy level (1 to 5) (1 lowest and 5 highest)	

Yoga Practice Record

Please practice yoga every day and after the practice mark your progress in the record below.

Practice record Week 9 to 12

Week 9	Sun	Mon	Tue	Wed	Thu	Fri	Sat
Yoga Practice							
Week 10	Sun	Mon	Tue	Wed	Thu	Fri	Sat
Yoga Practice							
Week 11	Sun	Mon	Tue	Wed	Thu	Fri	Sat
Yoga Practice							
Week 12	Sun	Mon	Tue	Wed	Thu	Fri	Sat
Yoga Practice							

After week 12 what improvement do you feel, please write in the box below

Wellness Monitor

Well done now you have completed 12 week of yoga practice, please take couple of minutes to fill in the following wellness monitor.

	Wellness Monitor	
S.N.	Indicators	After 12 week
1	Blood Pressure (High)	
	(Low)	
2	Lower back pain	
3	Shoulder Pain	
4	Neck Pain	
5	Quality of sleep (1 to 5) (1 lowest and 5 the best, average for the week)	
6	Stress level (1 to 5) (1 lowest and 5 highest, average for the week)	
7	Overall energy level (1 to 5) (1 lowest and 5 highest)	

Glossary

Spine

Spine is a series of interlocking bones called vertebrae and supported by muscles and ligaments.

The spine is affected by every movement of the body as it is attached to our arms by shoulders, our legs via pelvis and chest via ribs. So if our posture is not correct while sitting, lifting weight, etc then it is bound to affect our spine. Similarly if our joints are stiff (*which are attached to the spine*) then our spine will be more affected whenever they move. So for a healthy spine we need to have a correct posture and flexibility.

Natural curves of the spine:

Cervical (Neck)

Thoracic (Upper back)

Lumbar (Lower Back)

Natural curves of the spine are important as they allow the spine to act as a shock absorber. Too much or too little curve in any of the spine area can lead to pain. Our incorrect posture while sitting, jumping, etc effect our natural curve of the spine.

Vertebrae

The vertebrae are solid bones (roughly cylindrical) stack on one another and separated by the spinal disc. By nature the lumbar (lower back) vertebrae in our body are bigger as they take most of the load in our body and the cervical vertebrae are smaller as they take less of the load.

Spinal discs

The spinal discs are elastic tissues between vertebrae acting as cushions or shock absorbers and protect the spine from the impact from running, jumping, etc.

Facet Joints

The facet joints are at the back of the spine where one bone meets another bone. These joints prevent from overstretching your disc.

Spinal Nerves

The job of the spinal nerves is to carry messages to and fro from the brain.

Spinal Cord

A collection of nerves.

Sacroiliac Joints

SI joints are the links between the pelvis and the spine.

Pelvis

Pelvis joins the spine to the legs.

Osteoporosis

It is a loss of the bone minerals which results in thinning of the bone.

Reference:

(1) Back Care The Charity for Healthier Back, "Back Facts"<online> http://www.backpain.org/pages/b_pages/backfacts-2007.php

(2) American Chiropractic Association; Patients, "Back Pain Facts & Statistics" <online> http://www.amerchiro.org/level2_css.cfm?T1ID=13&T2ID=68

(3)Health and Safety Executive, HSE press release - 2 June 2005<online> http://www.hse.gov.uk/press/2005/e05077.htm

Dear Yoga Practitioner,

While practicing yoga exercises if you come across any question, you are welcome to send us your query at: info@subodhgupta.com

More information about us is available at

www.subodhgupta.com

You are also welcome to send us your experience about managing backache with the help of yoga if you would like them to be published on our website.

I wish you good health and happiness in your life.

With Best Regards
Subodh Gupta

Workshops and Yoga classes at workplace in London

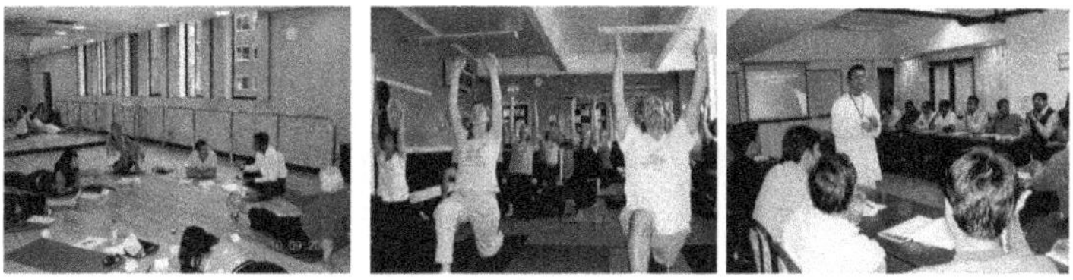

We provide following workshops and yoga classes for corporate organizations and Celebrities in London.

(1)Private Yoga sessions for Golfers/ Celebrities

(2) Half hour/ One hour Yoga Workshops for rejuvenation during day long Conferences and board meetings

(3)4 hours workshop on Work Life Balance / Stress Management

(4) 6 week Weight Management program for Celebrities

For more details please contact:

Barbara Tomasik
Indian Foundation for Scientific Yoga and Stress Management
44(0)7966275913 (London)
info@subodhgupta.com, barbara@subodhgupta.com

www.subodhgupta.com

Our Published books

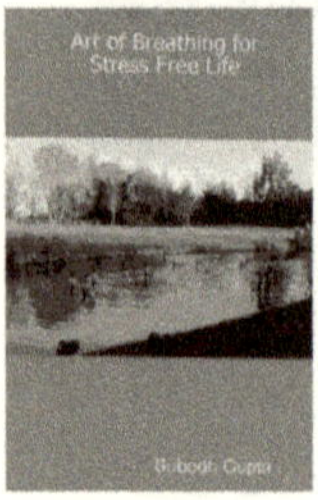

Art of Breathing *for* Stress free Life

The Only book on human breathing techniques for managing stress with clearly illustrated photographs and practical instructions. This book is ideal for busy people who lead a hectic life style.

Paperback/£4.95/ 56 pages

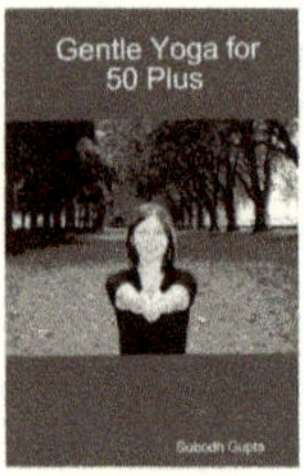

Gentle Yoga for 50 Plus

"A perfect gift of health for your parents"

The only book on Gentle Yoga for people in the age group of 50 plus. The exercises explained in this book are also beneficial if suffering from arthritis or rheumatism.

Paperback/ £5.95/ 68 pages

All our books are available at Amazon, Barnes and Nobles

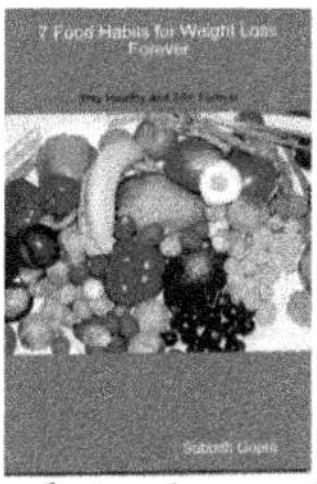

7 Food Habits for Weight Loss *Forever*

Stay Healthy and Slim *Forever*

"For anybody who wants to lose weight and gain health forever"

"Managing perfect body weight is not a complicated rocket science. Our body is made up of food which we eat during our day to day life. If we are overweight or obese at the moment then one thing is certain that the food which we eat is not good."

Healthy Food Habits = Good Health + Perfect Body Weight *Forever*

ISBN 978-0-9556882-0-1
Page 68 / Soft Cover / £4.95

Stress Management A Holistic Approach

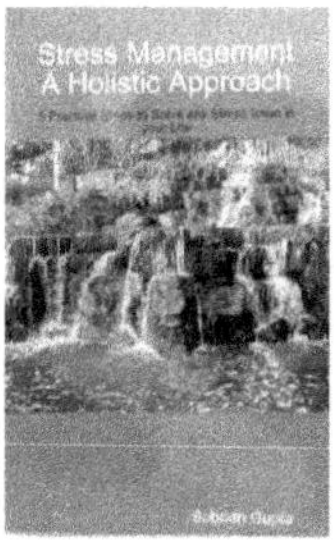

5 steps plan to manage Stress in your life

Many illnesses such as diabetes, migraine, asthma, ulcer and even cancer arise because of excessive Stress over the period of time.

You may have any kind of problem or issue in your life, once you follow the 5 steps described in this book you are on your way to Stress free life. If there is a problem then there has to be a solution and this book is all about solution.

ISBN 978-0-9556882-1-8
Page 80 / Soft Cover / £4.95

All our books are also available at Amazon.com, Barnes and Nobles

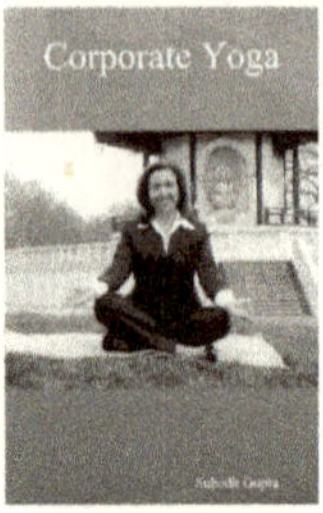

Corporate Yoga

"The Only Book on Corporate Yoga"

This simplified book of corporate yoga has been written considering the need of people working in the corporate sector.

This book will help in relieving pain from lower back, neck, fingers and forearms. It will also help in making eye muscles stronger, releasing stress and keeping the blood pressure normal.

ISBN 978-0-9556882-2-5
Page 96 / Soft Cover / £19.95

Simplified Yoga for Golfers

The yoga plan in this book is carefully designed for people who play golf.

A strong and flexible body creates the foundation for injury-free golf game. Simplified Yoga poses described in this book will not only strengthen the muscles but will also help to bring flexibility.

Flexibility + Strength = Injury - free Golf Game

ISBN 978-0-9556882-3-2
Page 96 / Soft Cover / £24.95

For more details please visit our website:
www.subodhgupta.com/books.html

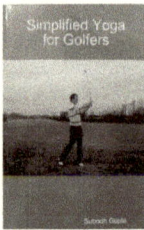

India Culture and Travel scams

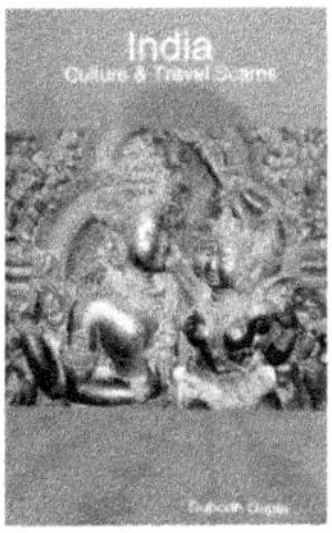

"The only book on travel scams targeted at western tourists in India"

This is a practical book about understanding Indian culture and travel scams in India and is based on real life experiences.

This book will help you to avoid embarrassing mistakes and prepare you to feel confident in unfamiliar situations.

Content in this book includes Indian social customs, their perception about Western women, their religion, what motivates them, travel scams targeted at Western tourists and of course what not to discuss with Indians, etc.

Page 112/Paper Back / £5.95
ISBN 978-0-9556882-6-3

For more details please visit our website:
www.subodhgupta.com/books.html

All our books are available at Amazon.com, Amazon.co.uk, Barnes and Nobles, Waterstones, WH Smith and Borders.

www.ingramcontent.com/pod-product-compliance
Lightning Source LLC
Chambersburg PA
CBHW022131280326
41933CB00007B/639
* 9 7 8 0 9 5 5 6 8 8 2 4 9 *